Shed Weight by Fasting

A comparison of the most popular fasting cures

From therapeutic fasting after Buchinger up to base fasting

Dr. Matt Roberts

Published by:

JoelNoah S.A.

info@joelnoah.com

Author: Dr. Matt Roberts

Shed Weight by Fasting - A comparison of the most popular fasting cures

From therapeutic fasting after Buchinger up to base fasting

ISBN-13: 978-1493747443

ISBN-10: 1493747444

Edition License Notes

TABLE OF CONTENTS

Attention

If you are taking medication for high cholesterol, high blood pressure, or diabetes, then please consult your doctor about the food products mentioned in this book. Your cholesterol level, high blood pressure, and diabetes should be naturally remedied! It is possible that you will no longer need your medications.

Should you be on the lookout for topics relating to health and medicine, you will find numerous books under my name in renowned bookstores.

Introduction

Therapeutic fasting is a conscious renunciation of solid foods, alcohol and tobacco for a specific period. Therapeutic fasting wasn't originally designed for health reasons, but for ethical and religious purposes. This is why the Catholics observe a fast between Lent and Easter.

Therapeutic fasting is a good opportunity to take time for yourself and free your body of "burdens" and, as a side effect - desirable for many - lose excess weight. Constant malnutrition, often combined with excessive alcohol or smoking, in the long-term leads to bioaccumulation in the body. The consequence is that you feel listless and incapable, or you can even suffer from mental disorders and later become ill.

During the therapeutic fast, value is placed on a lot of liquid intake, regular bowel evacuation, strolls out in the fresh air, and rest periods. Not only are bodily functions enhanced, but the mind and the soul while be "purified" and often get a glimpse of new experiences.

Everybody can choose from the different types of therapeutic fast to find one that meets their needs.

With a therapeutic fast, men can lose up to 6 kg (13 lbs) in 10 days of fasting, and women can lose 5 Kg (11 lbs).

Overview

Therapeutic Fasting - How Often and How Long

The question of fast frequency and duration does not have one all-inclusive answer. It depends on the starting situation, state of health, motivation, and of course the discipline that can be applied. Overall, 1 to 2 fasts per year are definitely recommended.

Therapeutic fasting can serve as an introduction to a long-term adjustment of living habits and nourishment. This especially applies if weight is lost from fasting. 1 to 2 fasts per year does not show any long-term success, if the person keeps feasting the way they are used to. With long-term dietary adjustments, additional fasts become superfluous.

Based on the respective duration, you should pay attention to how your body feels. The body signals when it needs more nourishment. Overall, a therapeutic fast of 5-14 days is recommended. Regular fasts, which allow for nourishment in small amounts, can be carried out longer than fasts with almost absolute abrosia - at least for the untrained.

Basically you should not stick so closely to recommendations - they can be nothing more than general guidelines based on experience. The human being is an individual with their own needs, and these should be accommodated. If the fast just feels torturous, it makes little sense to continue "through hell or high water" because the fast has to be carried out for x-amount of days.

However, during a therapeutic fast, alleviation of chronic illnesses only occurs after 14 days. A therapeutic fast of 6-8 weeks can be prolonged for chronic illnesses. In that case, the fast should not be conducted of your own accord at home, but rather under a doctor's supervision. There are special therapeutic fasting clinics or convents which offer a support program along with their own fasts. In any event, the therapeutic fast gets easier in a group with like-minded people. Upon request, the doctor can administer additional nourishment or bring about the end of the fast.

Suitability of the Therapeutic Fast

Healthy people can carry out a therapeutic fast without any further ado. However, beforehand you should make a check-up appointment with your physician to be sure that there are no reasons to avoid a therapeutic fast. This especially applies for people who want to conduct a therapeutic fast at home. Gaining background knowledge is also important, because there are a few important points about therapeutic fasting which should be observed to prevent any damage to your health.

If there are health-related restrictions, a doctor's appointment should be made in advance to find the ideal fast with the doctor. For serious illnesses, it is definitely prudent to conduct a therapeutic fast in a special clinic. There you will find professional personnel who can watch over your state of health and intervene if necessary.

Individuals suffering from eating disorders like bulimia, anorexia nervosa, or hyperphagia should by no means start fasting. Psychological help can be provided in a clinic, which gives you the chance to relieve this disorder.

A therapeutic fast is not recommended for individuals who are already heavily malnourished or suffer from infirmity and anemia.

People who have been instructed to take medication must speak with their doctor about which fast is suitable for them, which would not disrupt the medication's effects or - because of the altered metabolism - cause reverse effects.

Pregnant women must abstain from fasting, because the infant organism is nourished by the expecting mother. This alone is already an extraordinary circumstance for the maternal organism, who should not be burdened any further. This also prevents possible malnourishment of the mother and child. Children and adolescents should stay away from fasting, as their bodies are still growing and should be consistently nourished with nutrients.

Seriously sick individuals such as those suffering from cancer, tuberculosis, or thyroid disorders should abstain from therapeutic fasting. This illnesses already drain on the body's substance, which would be worsened by nutrient restriction / abstention.

For illnesses like depression, psychoses, diabetes, and gout, a doctor should by all means be consulted in advance, as a fast is not entirely to be avoided but - based on individual health - it should be carried out in a special clinic.

For abscesses or chronic inflammation of the stomach, you should at least consult a doctor first.

People who have recently been operated on, or have gone through a severe infection, are generally still weakened. It all depends on the reason for the operation, procedure, etc., so that based on circumstances a therapeutic fast can be helpful, but a doctor should be consulted beforehand.

Effects of the Therapeutic Fast

The body cleans itself of bioaccumulation and toxins, so excess weight is reduced in short order. The skin shows fewer impurities, seems smoother and more taut, and skin colour gets rosier. Hair profits from the fast with more tone. The muscles and overall bodily tissues get tighter, so posture is improved. The immune system is strengthened. Mentally you feel at your peak and mood improves enormously. Sense of taste gets more acute.

Many sicknesses can be improved through fasting. These include aches in the back and small of the back, joint pains, headaches and migraines, loss of strength, depression, forgetfulness, nervousness, irritability, lack of sleep, allergies, atopic dermatitis, high blood pressure, blood clotting (arterial and venal), and others.

Help with Feelings of Hunger

For beginners, it may happen that feelings of hunger develop around the 3rd or 4th day. This is the body saying, "please feed me".

The organism knows two ways to generate energy. The

first way is the direct utilization of energy we take in while eating. The second way is the supply of energy from reserve depots. So we generally don't eat at night, and during the day, when we feel hungry, we don't always immediately have something edible prepared for us. However, energy is produced for us in this time. Between these two types of production, the body shifts its operations around based on need.

During the fast, we run exclusively on our reserves. Evacuating your bowels becomes of special importance: interestingly enough, no feelings of hunger arise with empty bowels. You should avoid using the masticatory muscles. By moving the masticatory muscles, the brain sends a message to the stomach saying, "Attention, food's on the way." So, when food fails to enter the stomach while you chew gum, the stomach starts to feel hungry.

In the first days of a therapeutic fast, it is advised to stay away from people who are eating, restaurants, cafés, cafeterias, etc. As long as the "savings program" of energy production is turned on, it doesn't make a difference to observe people eating and just drink tea or water yourself. It might also help to choose a time to fast when there are no special occasions, such as holidays.

A lot of liquids should be drunk during the day, it's best not to wait until you feel thirsty. Because thirst only arises when the body already urgently needs water. Drinks containing sweeteners should by no means be consumed, because sweeteners cause feelings of hunger.

Help with Halitosis

During the therapeutic fast, you may experience halitosis. Not everybody is affected by this, smokers more often than non-smokers. The smell is a result of the detoxification, and in this case the body is cleansing itself of toxins through mucous.

Measures against this include lots of tooth-brushing, and brushing the tongue, and use of mouthwash.

A sufficient amount of liquids helps dispel the toxins through urine, but if too little is drunk, then it results in a stronger segregation of it in the mouth's mucous membranes.

Sucking on lemon wedges temporarily improves breath, so drinking water can be enriched with lemon juice.

While moving around in the fresh air, it helps to inhale through the nose and exhale through the mouth.

Help Against Freezing

The body temperature sinks by a few tenths of a degree Celsius during a therapeutic fast. The body's cells nourish themselves with the body's reserves, the metabolism running on the "savings program". This causes shivering or freezing. This is entirely normal. You can help yourself with a few little tricks.

Even though a therapeutic fast can be carried out at any time, it is much more convenient to start the fast during a warmer time of year to combat the cold.

If the day starts out with a contrast shower, it promotes circulation and increases cutaneous perfusion - blood being delivered to the skin. If the skin is also rubbed with a brush or a luffa, this also increases cutaneous perfusion and greatly enhances the detoxification process.

Bodily movement also promotes circulation, so it is not important which particular sport you play. It should just be something fun, and which is not strongly based on performance.

Drinking hot tea warms the body from the inside. Fennel or ginger tea are especially good at warming the body.

Warm clothing always helps against the cold.

A hot foot bath can alleviate internal freezing.

Lying comfortably on the couch around noon or in the evening with a warm, cozy blanket can be a small wonder.

A hot-water bottle or a hot grain pillow cause the body to feel warm.

Visiting a Sauna

Sessions at a sauna are desirable during a fast, because it allows for detoxification through the skin.

If someone is fasting for the first time, or has never visit a sauna before, they should avoid visiting a sauna.

It should be observed that circulation reacts more sensitively than "normal". So you should not spend longer than normal in temperatures higher than 70° C (158° F). In temperatures up to 70° C, your stay can be carried out longer in peace. You should pay attention to when your body feels that it has had enough. Cooling off should also occur carefully and gently.

Effectiveness of "The Pill"

During the fast, the balance of hormones gets mixed up. Regardless of whether you take the Pill, it can result in early menstruation, or menstruation can skip a month, or two can occur one after the other.

The effectiveness of the Pill is questionable, partially because of the urgently required bowel evacuations during the fast. If you want to be careful to not become pregnant, then additional contraception should be used, such as condoms.

Gall Stones from a Therapeutic Fast?

You often hear about gall stones forming during a therapeutic fast. Rest assured, this is nonsense.

Gall stones mainly form from accumulation of cholesterol and crystalized waste products from the gall bladder. Because no nourishment is taken throughout the fast - and thus no fat - no gall stones form during the fast.

But it could happen that gall bladder waste has already formed before the fast. Then it would not be good to keep the gall bladder from working during the therapeutic fast, because the avoidance of fat and the inactive gall bladder could let the waste harden into stones.

If you are up to date on your high cholesterol level, this can be remedied by drinking gall bladder-promoting herbal tea. When it comes to herbs, the following should be considered: artichokes, blessed thistle, white fringetree, milk thistle, peppermint, radish, chamomile, sage, yarrow, candytuft, common centaury, and woodruff.

The Types of Therapeutic Fast

The most important types of fast will be described below. The most detailed is a description of Buchinger / Lützner, because this fast is one of the most common in practice. It contains overall guidelines that are applicable for all types of fast, such as days of relaxation; bowel cleansing; avoidance of alcohol, cigarettes, coffee; playing sports during the fast; quiet breaks; and days for developing your body.

Fasting by Dr. Otto Buchinger / Lützner

Buchinger was a German doctor whose teachings describe taking at least 5 days of voluntarily avoiding solid food. A low-calorie intake in the form of fruit or vegetable juice occurs, to supply the body with minerals and vitamins, and protein (if necessary) through dairy products. Daily calorie intake amounts to around 250 - 500 kcal.

An important element of the therapeutic fast is bowel evacuation, whereby the body is freed from contaminants and toxic substances which have accumulated in the body from poor nourishment or the metabolism.

Self-regulating forces are activated. But the toxic substances are also segregated through the kidneys and skin.

If the intestine is fully emptied, then feelings of hunger rarely arise during the therapeutic fast. Liquid intake is extremely important, because detoxification through the kidneys is only possible with a sufficient amount of healthy liquids. The daily required amount is at least 2.5 L or, put in other terms: around 0.2 L per hour.

Throughout the therapeutic fast, especially in the first days, there can be some undesired side-effects such as fatigue, headaches, or sluggish limbs. But don't let this discourage you. This is a sign that the body has begun the detoxification process. Harmful substances which have accumulated over a long period of time, oftentimes over decades, are now being expelled in large amounts and circulate in the blood flow until they are released. These symptoms will ease after a few days. Should the symptoms not weaken, then visiting a doctor is recommended.

Headaches can be caused by too meager liquid intake or too little movement, too much stress or too rare bowel evacuations. Heavy coffee drinkers can experience withdrawal, but this gives way after 1-2 days. It is helpful to successively reduce coffee consumption 1-2 weeks before starting the fast.

Normally the Buchinger fast begins with 2 days of relief. This means that a few days before the fast begins, you prepare by only ingesting easily digestible food such as fruit, vegetables, natural yoghurt, sometimes rice, etc. That way, initiating the fast is not so difficult (reduction of calorie intake), and the body then already starts detoxification and is not overloaded with waste. Plus the person fasting becomes mentally prepared for the upcoming purification.

A purification of the intestines occurs on the first day of the fast. For this, discharge agents like Glauber salt, Epsom salt, F. X. Passage SL powder, or other over-the-counter compounds should be considered. Enemas are also suitable, and can come in handy.

After that, you may only drink: fruit or vegetable juices may be drunk, preferably diluted with regular mineral water. Unlimited amounts of mineral water. You can support certain organ systems with herbal teas, such as the kidneys, to expel more harmful substances. There are also fasting teas which generally activate the detoxification organs. When necessary, the tea can be slightly sweetened with honey; sugar and sweeteners are not useful.

A vegetable roth is expedient, as it supports the organism's deacidification. However, powdered soups or instant vegetable stocks are taboo. They contain too much salt and most also contain botanically hydrogenated fats which harm the body. Flavour enhancers within, like glutamate, arouse the appetite. You should take the time to make a stock out of fresh (root) vegetables. The broth fulfills the function of an alkaline counterweight, because lots of acids can be released while fasting, especially in the first days. Celery, carrots, and leeks are convenient. The vegetables are cut to small pieces and lightly simmered for a few hours. Then you strain the solid pieces through a sieve and only drink the broth.

A caloric intake of 500 kcal. should not be exceeded, because then the organism will switch to its normal metabolism.

The fast should be accompanied by light sports. For one, this promotes the deacidification process, and secondly sports prevent excessive muscle deterioration. Ideal sports are aqua jogging, meditative gymnastics, or even light gymnastics or walking.

If you engage in athletics every day anyway, this should fit well into your schedule. For endurance sports, you should consult a doctor. However, you should take care to strive for a performance increase in this time.

After 2 days at most, the intestine should be cleansed as described above. Digestive residue from the intestinal loops has "slid down" and the digestion of the body's reserves also creates waste products which have to be expelled, as well as water-insoluble waste. Myriad cells in our bodies die every day this way to make place for new cells. Now the intestine has less work, and it becomes sluggish based on the intestinal motor function and so has to receive a little push from the outside (see measures for bowel evacuation on Day 1).

In a special fasting clinic, additional offers are made in the form of massages, liver packs, etc., which help the body cleanse itself of waste.

When fasting at home, sauna visits are not only allowed, but recommended, provided you can generally seek out a sauna for health reasons.

Ending the fast (breaking the fast) must occur gently. All of the digestive organs are no longer used to carrying out their functions, and they have to slowly become reacquainted with their tasks.

It's best to begin the first two meals with an apple, well chewed. With the third meal, a small potato-vegetable soup is recommended. This should be prepared with fresh ingredients and ingested in small portions, because the appetite is not as strong as it was before the fast. Salt should be avoided, and herbs can be eaten without hesitation, through fresh herbs are preferable. A little glass of milk can be drunk now as well. The portions are slowly increased, to slowly reacquaint the body with solid food.

Symptoms of constipation can arise, which can be easily alleviated by ingesting digestion-promoting fruits such as prunes, kiwis, or fresh pineapple. Meals can be enriched by crisp bread with low-fat curd, with fresh herbs like chives or cress. The longer the fast lasted, the longer the restructuring days should take. A longer restructuring time prevents the yo-yo effect on the weight that was lost.

After that, virtually anything can be eaten again. You should make sure that your recently cleansed body is not soon overladen with toxins again. Whoever lost weight so bravely should try to maintain their new weight. A dietary change which is both sustainably healthy and low in calories would now be helpful. Whoever had weight loss as a priority and generally enjoys eating sweets will notice that their sense of taste has changed in favour of a more intensive perception. The desire for sweets will not initially be present. You should not fall back into old habits, otherwise the success of the fast is quickly nullified.

With the therapeutic fast, you can lose up to 1 kg (2.2 lbs) in the first few days, and eventually an average of 400-500 g (about 1 lbs)per day, around 100 g (0.22 lbs) less for women. This means that a man can lose 6 kg (13 lbs) of weight during a 10-day fast, and a woman can lose 5.2 kg (11 lbs). Now and again, losing weight will come to a standstill. Although calories are hardly taken in, you still don't lose weight. This is normal, and you should not be discouraged because after 1-2 days, the weight loss continues.

Fasting by Franz Xaver Mayr

This fast does not only consist of drinks, but also traditionally of around 2 days of old white flour / spelt flour biscuits. They should not be fresh by any means, but they should also be able to be broken down by the intestines. Each individual bite should be chewed for so long that it turns into an almost liquidy mass, and that a sweet taste comes about by the enzymes breaking down the carbohydrates. Before swallowing, you take a sip of milk and chew everything well again. When a feeling of fullness sets in, the meal is over. In the morning and evening, a 30 g (0.066 lbs) portion of lean cheese (like mozzarella or tofu) is allowed. This allows for protein intake to reduce muscle deterioration. If you desire, a clear vegetable broth can be had for lunch. Water and tea can be drunk throughout the day as desired.

With this fast, the stomach and the intestine are massively relieved of any burden. That is why this fast is especially suited for people with chronic digestive problems or stomach inflammation. A tolerance for milk and/or milk products is required for the successful diet. Alternatively, soy/rice/oat/coconut milk can be substituted.

People who already exhibit symptoms of deficiency should avoid this fast.

The F. X. Mayr diet is based around 4 pillars (= 4 S): **Sparing**, **Sanitation**, **Schooling** and **Substitution**.

Sparing is about moderation in the detoxification of the digestive organs, but also in the sense of replenishing inner peace through relaxation.

Sanitation concerns intestinal cleansing, whereby purging and deacidification are promoted with help from cleansing salts. But the other excretory organs' activities are enhanced - kidneys, skin, and respiration, for example. Enemas help with persistent constipation. The special thing about the F. X. Mayr diet is medicinal treatment of the torso (massage).

Schooling encompasses the training of proper chewing, a drink between meals - but never while eating -, general drink training, avoiding any distraction while eating, and learning proper eating habits.

With the **Substitution** of vitamins, dietary minerals, and mineral substances, as well as ingestion of base powders, deficiency symptoms are avoided with uniform nourishment.

Modern F. X. Mayr Diet

The F. X. Mayr diet has developed since Mayr's time. Due to the most diverse burdens, individual concept are necessary to be suitable for each person. So the therapy spectrum was enormously expanded to offer a unique solution for certain sicknesses. A prior examination and diagnosis are thus a part of the F. X. Mayr diet. It entails an assessment of the skin, hair, nails, posture, shape of the stomach, stomach constitution, but blood pressure is also measured, and lap parameters (blood levels) are pinpointed, among others.

So people with chronic illnesses can also join in on enjoying a therapeutic fast. If you appreciate a doctor's accompaniment, the therapeutic fast, like if you are chronically sick, the therapeutic fast can only occur through a special clinic.

Juice Fast

The juice fast can only be carried out with fruit and vegetable juice, and water. The body receives vitamins, minerals and mineral elements from the juices, plus a small amount of calories.

If you have a sensitive stomach or heartburn, vegetable juice should take priority over fruit juice because vegetable juices contain less acid and are thus better received. The perfect juice fast is done with raw juice. 750 ml of raw juice are drunk per day, divided into 3 "portions", preferably diluted with water.

Detoxification and deacidification can also be supported by freshly pressed plant juices (from the health store). You can also check to see which organ systems need support and choose the plant juices accordingly. Overall, the following mixture has proven true: 2 tablespoons of artichoke juice, 2 tablespoons of stinging nettle juice, and 4 tablespoons of potato juice mixed in together, ingested in the morning and evening.

Fasting with Protein

The special thing about this diet is that the body receives a certain amount of protein per day, which contain all essential amino acids.

To this end, various products are sold on the market as protein shakes. The Ulmer Drink or Almased® is rightfully popular. These are powders which are stirred into water or milk, and so can be considered a complete "meal".

Muscle deterioration can be prevented by this protein intake, and the body gets toned. The muscles are strongly driven by metabolism, and if they are built up, the resting metabolic rate loses energy. If you ingest protein, the resting metabolic rate stays level (like in the "normal state" with nourishment), and the loss of balance is accelerated because the body pulls directly from the fat reserves.

Whey Fasting

A typical day during a whey fast starts with a bowel cleanse. This is done by drinking a glass of sauerkraut or plum juice (around 0.2 l). Throughout the rest of the day you drink 1 l of whey. The protein it contains reduced muscle deterioration, and whey has a positive effect on the skin. To ensure supplication of minerals, vitamins, and energy, you also drink 0.5 l of fruit juice. Washing out toxins is done by an additional 3 l of non-carbonated mineral water.

Tea Fasting

Tea fasting is an extreme form of fast. This type should only be done by completely healthy people.

It is practically a zero diet, because only tea and water are drunk. Plain water is preferable, although barely carbonated water could be an alternative if necessary.

When selecting teas, there are special types which are meant to support specific organs or support fasting. You can find out more about these in pharmacies, because that is where the ingredients in teas are standardized, not in the supermarket.

This diet is especially designed to purge and detoxicate. But weight loss will also be quickly seen.

Schroth Diet

This diet is attributed to Johann Schroth. It entails a constant alternation between drinking days and dry days. On a dry day, you drink little and eat "stale rolls" and biscuits. On a drinking day, ingestion of liquids is the priority. Schroth recommended drinking a liter of red wine per day.

This type of fast is no longer practical, because we know that lots of liquids are required for detoxification and purging. Alcohol strains the liver and the weight-loss effect is reduced because alcohol is rich in calories.

Base Fasting

Base fasting in the narrow sense of the term is not a fast, but rather primarily serves for deacidification. For the duration of 1-2 weeks, exclusively basic (of a base) foodstuffs may be consumed. Excessive acids are ruled out.

The foundation of nourishment while base fasting are nearly all types of fruit and vegetables. With this low concentration of nutrients, it is possible to shed a few excess pounds.

A cool effect is the expulsion of acids from the body, whereas an over-acidification certainly occurs with "normal" eating. You should actually ingest about 80% of basic products and 20% acidic, although experience shows that this distribution is reversed.

deacidification causes detachment of the body fat. With base fasting, the following items are prohibited: meat, fish, eggs, dairy, sweets, coffee and black tea, alcohol, cigarettes, and grains (including rice and noodles).

This diet is especially suitable if you experience typical symptoms of over-acidification, such as fatigue and faintness, decreased motivation. Some sicknesses are tied in with over-acidification such as allergies, connective tissue weakness, intestinal illnesses, gout, hormonal disruptions, infections, headaches, osteoporosis and rheumatism. Over-acidification often causes a deficiency of minerals, even though they are ingested in large amounts through food. This is because the body tries to neutralize the acids with the minerals.

The base fast can be effectively enhanced with tissue

salts. This can prevent occasional side-effects of the fast like headaches - a result of detoxification - or at least alleviate them. Tissue salts act as a balanced mineral substitute.

Porridge Fasting

People with extremely sensitive stomachs or intestines are well-suited for the porridge fast. With this diet, you only ingest grain puree from various types of grain like rice, oatmeal and buckwheat.

The advantage of this diet lies in its supply of protein and carbohydrates. Muscles do not deteriorate, and you always get full. Weight is lost, with no yo-yo effect.

The disadvantage, however, is the soggy taste and texture, and it rarely leads to detoxification and/or purging.

For the porridge fast, a plate of oat porridge is eaten three times per day for a week. You should also move around a lot.

A multi-day porridge fast can be used as a relief day before entering another fast. This way, normal nourishment is interrupted and the body can tune itself to the upcoming restrictions.

Breuss Diet

This diet was developed by Rudolf Breuss, an Austrian holistic practitioner. It is designed for cancer patients who take 42 days avoiding solid food and only ingest certain juices and types of tea.

The goal is to starve cancer cells which require lots of protein. The theory states that cancer cells consist of protein and are broken down by this fast.

Carrying out this diet is recommended in a special clinic, because doctor supervision can be given here. This is an important aspect for such a serious condition and its potential danger.

Juices are used in this diet, primarily consisting of red and yellow turnips, celery, radish and - based on the type of cancer - potato juice. When fasting at home, the juice can be acquired from the pharmacy.

The most important drink in the Breuss diet is sage tea. Storksbill tea helps patients who have already gone through radiation.

A day with the Breuss diet can go like this: a half-cup of tea for the kidneys in the morning, with sage tea an hour later; this can be enriched with peppermint or lemon balm. After another hour, the Breuss juice can be drank in small sips. Overall, the maximum daily amount of the vegetable juice comes to a half liter.

Through noon and the afternoon, kidney tea is drunk again. The Breuss diet also supposedly combats cancer prophylactically, purifying the blood and alleviating joint pain. Playing sports and keeping the mind active support this diet and should distract the patient from their illness.

The diet is problematic for people whose immune system has been severely impaired.

The Breuss diet is not scientifically recognized, although there are many reports from people who were hopeless cases to academic medicine and were cured by the Breuss diet.

Fasting by Hildegard von Bingen

This fast is very old. Hildegard von Bingen lived during the Middle Ages and was active in naturally healing sick people, among other things. Along with bodily cleansing, mental reflection is of central importance. At the end of the fast, you should feel more vivaciousness and a better mood.

The fast begins with a preparation period, wherein there is a gentle bowel evacuation. For instance, Hildegard von Bingen recommended ginger pellets.

The fast occurs in three stages. In the first phase, spelt products (spelt porridge, spelt bread) and fruits and vegetables may be ingested. Water and fennel tea are drunk in addition to this. This lasts for 1-2 days. In the next phase, spelt-vegetable broth is consumed for up to 5 days. In the third phase, reconstruction of nourishment of the usual fare begins for 1-2 days. Extending the reconstruction period is certainly beneficial.

Soup Fasting

The soup fast is intended for people who are thin - for whom weight loss is not a real priority, but rather cleansing, purging, and deacidification.

The soup fast lasts for 3 days. The first day of the fast begins with a breakfast of 2-3 small apples, which are eaten throughout the morning. On the second and third days, there is only unsweetened tea and water in an unlimited amount.

A fast soup is eaten for lunch. It is best to make it fresh, i.e. from a small amount (around 200 g or 0.44 lbs) of potatoes (or spelt), a half bunch of soup vegetables, 1 bulb of fennel, your preferred herbs and 1 l of water. The vegetables are cut small and cooked with the water for half an hour. Finally the soup is strained through a sieve, presented, and drank.

There is more fast soup in the evening. Lots of fluids are drunk throughout the day and - as with all fasts - cleansing the intestine and skin, movement, and breaks of solitude are crucial.

Conclusion

Healthy people have a large range of therapeutic fasts to choose from. Sick people should figure out with their doctor which therapeutic fast is best for them immediately before starting their fast.

Regardless of which type you choose, success will happen. This includes losing weight in a short time, you will be amazed at your spiritual health and the ease with which you carry out your daily tasks.

When it comes to weight loss, people profit most when they adjust their eating habits after fasting and avoid typical calorie bombs.

www.ingramcontent.com/pod-product-compliance
Lightning Source LLC
Chambersburg PA
CBHW070940290526
45795CB00003B/1090